HCG DIET COOKBOOK

Top 50 Delicious Chinese-American HCG Diet Recipes

TABLE OF CONTENTS

Introduction

I want to thank you and congratulate you for purchasing the book *HCG Diet Cookbook: Top 50 Delicious Chinese-American HCG Diet Recipes*.

The HCG diet requires dedication to a simple but specific protocol, and you've taken a great step by downloading this book. It may seem daunting at first, but following the plan can be easy, cost-effective, and delicious. Through the integration of these recipes into your diet, you'll see fast and dramatic changes in your weight.

This book contains an abundance of delicious and classic Chinese-American recipes that adhere to the approved HCG food list. Recipes are provided for all meals of the day, making it easy to eat healthy all day, every day. The primary focus is placed on simple, cost-effective ingredients that you can find at most grocery stores. All recipes use basic cooking techniques, equipment, and appliances, meaning that these will be very accessible to home chefs. Note that all recipes are for a single serving unless otherwise noted. You'll need to use these recipes within your larger HCG strategy, understanding what counts for your protein or vegetable serving.

For these recipes, feel free to make minor substitutions if you have an allergy. Understanding what the purpose of an ingredient is in a recipe will help you understand what a good substitute may be. Talk to your physician if you need more guidance or if you have other issues such as diabetes. Additionally, it's widely recognized that frozen fruits and vegetables are just as nutritious as fresh versions, so please feel free to swap in a frozen option if it seems appropriate.

The first and most important step towards losing weight is recognizing that you want to see change and then committing yourself to taking action. You've made it so far, and for that, congratulations.

Thank you very much again for downloading this book.

Chapter 1

The HCG Diet Overview

If you're reading this book, you probably already know the basic concepts and protocol of the HCG diet plan. The plan combines a very low-calorie, high-protein, high-vegetable cleanse with the benefits of a human chorionic gonadotropin (HCG) supplement. These supplements come in the form of injections, pills, or drops. HCG is naturally produced by the body during pregnancy, and the use of an HCG supplement by dieters is said to actually reset the timing of your metabolism, leading to quick weight loss. Moreover, the HCG will actually suppress hunger, meaning you won't even feel hungry.

Many HCG diet plans either have three or four total phases. All plans typically have a first phase where dieters are asked to load up on fattening food and feast on large meals. The basis of this is to stock the body's fat reserves as much as possible before cutting to so few calories. The idea is that you must gain before losing.

The primary and longest phase of the HCG diet is the second phase where dieters take the HCG hormone and carry through with the low-calorie portion of the plan. Dieters typically take two meals a day, each of which consists of 100 grams of meat, a vegetable, a fruit, and a slice of bread. Consuming more whole foods, such as vegetables and fruits, is a fantastic way of nourishing your body and losing weight. No visible fats on the meat are allowed; extra fat must be removed! Butter, oils, and fats cannot be used in cooking. Fattier fish are typically not allowed in the diet either. You can, however, take as much water, coffee, or tea as desired. Lemon juice is allowed but only one lemon's worth. Milk can be added but only a single tablespoon's worth. No sugar is allowed to sweeten drinks, but sugar substitutes are allowed. Vinegar (apple cider), mustard powder, sea salt, pepper, and spices can be added to dishes as well. The second chapter of the book will provide a handy list of what foods are typically accepted as part of the diet.

Note that it's absolutely possible to carry out the HCG diet while being a vegetarian or vegan. You can get all required nutrients from a plant-based diet. Feel free to substitute any meat specified in the recipes with an equal amount of tofu, tempeh, or pulses, if you feel comfortable doing so. Eggs and cottage cheese have also been used successfully as alternatives. Plant-based protein shakes made with water are also an excellent substitute for meat.

The third and possibly fourth phases involve ending the HCG hormone supplements and slowly introducing more calories into your diet. This phase is important in acclimating to a normal diet once again. By the end, the dieter's metabolism should be altered as to maintain weight loss for the long term.

The traditional diet limits you to 500 calories a day, although many modern versions allow many more calories than that. Whichever form of the diet you choose is up to you. We'll just provide you with the recipes to help you stick with your plan!

Here are our top 20 tips to help you stay true to the HCG diet:

1. Remember to stay hydrated! Drinking adequate amounts of water will help your body feel fuller and make it a little more tolerable when you're eating less food. Also, water helps keep your muscles feeling energized, which is a big concern of many people on the HCG diet. Muscle fatigue can result when your body's cells don't maintain a proper balance of fluid. Staying well-hydrated means that your body will move around all of the nutrients in the body, digest food properly, and stay properly cooled or heated. Switch between water and tea to keep things fresh. Tea is a classic

3

component of the Chinese meal, and many claim that a cup of hot tea helps digestion.

2. Stevia is an amazing invention. While on the HCG diet, stevia can help you keep your sugar cravings at bay. Additionally, many different flavored varieties of stevia exist, including vanilla, toffee, chocolate, lemon, root beer, orange, and so many more. A lot of the recipes in this book use a packet of stevia to add a touch of sweetness, which is a characteristic in Chinese-American cuisine! If you'd like to use an appropriate-flavored stevia when stevia is specified in a recipe (Orange Stevia for an Orange Chicken recipe), please feel free to do so. It's important to feel like you have options while on the HCG diet, as food boredom can definitely be an issue for some people. When purchasing stevia, remember to check the brand and list of ingredients. Not all stevias are made the same, and some may include fillers. Only purchase "pure" stevia, as that's the only type allowed on the HCG diet.

3. If you must make social plans at a restaurant, try to do some research on a restaurant that may have meal options for you, even if those options are limited to side dishes. Many restaurants offer a single vegetable side dish, such as a dish of spinach or broccoli. If you think these will be cooked with additional fats or oils, call ahead of time and check to see if they can just steam it for you. Additionally, some people even bring their own food ahead of time to the restaurant and request that they plate it for them to have a true dining experience. The restaurant will typically just charge for their least expensive item on the menu to offset the labor cost of serving it to you. Not all restaurants will do this, so make sure to check beforehand!

4. Save money by purchasing meat in bulk at the grocery store. Once you bring the meat home, prep everything at the same time, cutting portions, trimming fat, weighing amounts, and placing meat into plastic bags. Freeze for later use. If you're a talented meal planner,

you can also plan ahead your meals for the week. It's a huge timesaver and a huge money saver!

5. Make sure to get enough calories every day. Even if you don't feel hungry, make sure you reach the optimal calorie amount you're looking to achieve. Your body can easily feel sluggish, your brain can slow down, and your blood sugar can drop too low if you're not eating enough every day. This may not be an issue for some of you (many have no trouble reaching their maximum calories!), but just keep this in mind for the future.

6. Greens are a gift from the HCG gods. You can consume so many leafy green vegetables, such as spinach, lettuce, and Swiss chard, without worrying about calories. Most are very water-heavy, meaning that eating a lot of the greens will help you feel full. To top it off, these greens are packed with nutrients. There's an outdated concept that plain lettuce isn't very nutritious, but that's false. Lettuce and other greens are filled with vitamins, fiber, and trace minerals that you may have a hard time getting from other foods. In fact, a serving of spinach has half a day's worth of your Vitamin A! You can bulk eat salad greens and never have to worry about exceeding your calorie limit for the day. Compared to some other veggies, such as asparagus or onions, greens can be consumed in essentially unlimited amounts. Just be careful to have a good sense of how much dressing you consume with your greens. A light shake of salt and citrus juice can do wonders alone.

7. Bring food with you when you're on the go! Bring your fruit for the day as your snack, or if you have something prepared already, bring it with you to ensure you eat the right food. If you're working in an office, it can be easy to just go out for lunch with your coworkers. However, small mistakes and slip-ups can seriously throw off the HCG diet. You need to make sure you're prepared so that you can't find an excuse to go off the approved foods' list.

8. Keep the handbags of frozen vegetables that can be easily steamed in a microwave. These are especially handy to take to the office! Just bring a packaged bag of frozen vegetables with you every day and heat it up in the microwave. Keep a stash of spices on your desk and switch up the seasonings every day to keep things feeling fresh. Bring a cooked piece of protein to heat up on the side, and you have a full, healthy meal ready for the middle of the day.

9. Try not to think about food that's unacceptable to the HCG plan. It's difficult to stay on track when you're watching TV commercials and cooking shows that discuss all the delicious food you aren't allowed to eat! Try not to read too many non-HCG recipes. Eventually, once you're on the later phases, you can begin researching healthy, whole food recipes that allow more calories into your diet, without compromising your long-term weight loss goals.

10. Spread out your calorie allotments throughout the day, taking an early coffee or tea, your first meal at lunchtime, and your second meal at dinnertime. Spread out snacks in between. Keeping a regular meal schedule is a good way to stave off hunger, as your stomach will start to learn when to expect food and how much food to expect. You can also break up individual portions of food, such as the 1-bread portion for the day. Eat half a breadstick or piece of Melba toast in the morning and the other half in the middle of the day. Also, pay attention to when your eating should be restricted in relation to your HCG supplement. Many protocols specify that you shouldn't eat 15 to 30 minutes before or after taking HCG.

11. A lot of HCG dieters swear by gum! A good sugar-free gum can help control food cravings and manage hunger, thereby helping you stick to the HCG plan. Gum alone won't make the fat melt off; however, it could help a dieter stick to a thoughtful weight loss plan. Check the ingredients for the chewing gum of your choice to ensure that the artificial sweeteners are acceptable to the HCG plan.

12.   Protein shakes made with water can be an excellent way of satisfying a sweet tooth and getting your requisite protein for the day without going over on calories. Do some research to find one that fits your dietary needs, as there are a wealth of options out there. Not all protein powders are made alike; some have way too much sugar that is acceptable on the HCG diet, so you absolutely must decipher the ingredient list.

13.   Pickles! Surprisingly, pickles are very much acceptable to the HCG protocol. Most pickles have very little carbs and generally no fat. If you think about it, both cucumbers and vinegar are allowed as per the HCG acceptable foods list, and pickles are just cucumbers pickled in vinegar. This snack has an excellent and satisfying crunch, vinegary bite, and refreshing texture, making it a fantastic way to curb cravings. Note that pickles may have excess sugar or salt; however, so check the label to buy the best pickles possible.

14.   On that note, be careful of how much salt you add to your meals. It's easy to go overboard when you're directed to add sea salt to taste. The intention of "to taste" is to allow dieters to add no salt if they feel like it's flavorful enough already! As you reduce your salt intake, your flavor palette and body will get used to less salt in your meals. Reducing salt is an excellent way to reduce water retention in the body, meaning that at least in the short term, you'll see pounds shedding off quickly. Those extra pounds lost may be what you need to motivate yourself to stick with the diet!

15.   Stay on track by getting in touch with other HCG dieters online. The community is one of the fundamental pillars of human relationships, and being able to talk, ask questions to, support, cheer on, and commiserate with other dieters are enormously helpful. Find inspiration in others, and you'll be more motivated to keep going! Talk with your friends and family about your diet plan as well, and they'll be more cognizant of how to best support you. Be aware of what your emotional triggers are regarding food.

16.   Do your research on different HCG protocols. Many diet plans are out of date, and some are also just inaccurate. Many foods were not around in the 1950s when the initial research was being performed on the diet. By confirming that these foods are acceptable, you can open up a whole horizon of additional foods to consume during the second phase of the plan.

17.   Ensure that HCG products are purchased from reputable providers. Not all providers, especially on the Internet, can be considered trustworthy. Some hormones can be poor quality or even contaminated, and it's just not worth risking your health. Purchase hormones only from licensed, well-established providers. Get specific advice from their team medical staff regarding the suggested usage.

18.   Talk to a physician and nutritionist about your HCG diet plan. It's important to get a professional's opinion before starting any major diet strategy, and any major nutritional decisions should be made under the guidance of someone who knows your health history. A physician can monitor your blood work and health condition to make sure that the HCG diet is right for you.

19.   Get excited about healthy, whole foods! Research the health benefits of HCG diet, which only uses whole foods rather than processed foods. After you complete the HCG diet, try to maintain a diet of primarily whole foods with the occasional treat. Making food at home is a great strategy to achieve this. Weight loss occurs as a result of lifestyle changes, not a quick diet. That's why most diet plans simply don't work for the long term. Regardless of weight loss, research shows that whole foods, such as lentils, whole grains, fruits, and vegetables, have a major positive impact on your health. This may go unseen in that nutritious foods may prevent certain diseases and health issues, but your body and mind will also just feel good eating nutritious food. Many digestive issues can be solved by eating well. Your body will thank you.

20.   Find go-to recipes that you can make quickly and easily when you're tired at the end of the day, and you don't know what to eat. Hopefully, some of these delicious Chinese-American recipes will make it into your weekly rotation! Keep a list or planner of absolute-must, go-to recipes that you know will be quick and delicious. Having the required ingredients stocked in your kitchen will help with this. In the next chapter, we'll look at what foods are acceptable to the HCG diet. Try to have your favorites always stocked at home!

Chapter 2

Approved Food List

The HCG diet dictates a specific list of foods that can be consumed during the second phase of the plan. Keeping your refrigerator and pantry stocked with these whole foods is an easy way to make sure you're cooking with the right ingredients!

You may want to purchase a kitchen scale, as the protein portions for the second phase are exactly 100 grams. Having a scale to check the portion size will be immensely helpful. Additionally, after you've finished the HCG protocol, kitchen scales are a fantastic tool for baking and for portion control, so consider it a long-term investment in your kitchen arsenal.

Vegetables can generally be eaten in any amount, depending on the strictness of the HCG diet protocols followed. Just be sure to pay attention to the calorie content of the vegetables.

List of Approved Proteins:

- Lean beef
- Veal
- Lean chicken
- Whitefish
- Lobster
- Crab

- Shrimp

- Scallops

- Egg (1 whole) plus egg whites (3, or approximately 0.5 C.)

- Cottage cheese (fat-free)

- Tofu

- Tempeh

- Pulses (lentils, etc.)

Note that proteins cannot be cooked on the bone. Also, remember that pieces must be trimmed of all fat and skin.

List of Approved Vegetables:

- Chicory

- Spinach

- Onions

- Chard

- Cauliflower

- Fennel

- Celery

- Cucumbers

- Beet greens

- Mixed greens

- Cabbage

- Lettuce

- Red radishes

- Shallots
- Asparagus
- Broccoli
- Tomatoes

List of Approved Fruits:

- Strawberries
- Blueberries
- Raspberries
- Blackberries
- Cherries
- Lemons
- Apples
- Oranges
- Grapefruit

List of Approved Bread:

- Melba toast
- Breadsticks

Chapter 3

Soups and Salads

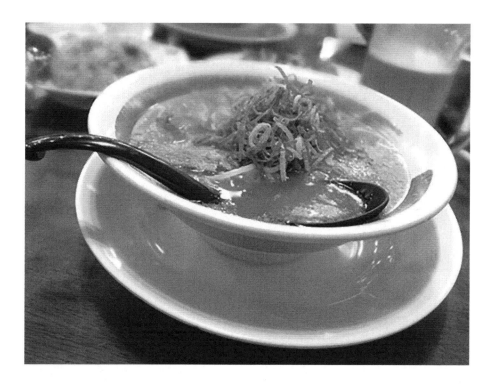

Chinese Scallion Soup

This soup is light and full of flavor! Scallions, also known as green onions, are a classic part of any Chinese dish, whether as a primary flavor component or just as a colorful garnish. Scallions have a good amount of Vitamin C and an exceptional amount of Vitamin K. Their onion flavor is mildly sweet and slightly less intense than other onion varietals. While many chefs use either the white end or the green end, this recipe will use the whole stalk of scallion. Extra pieces are added as a garnish on top, making this a truly beautiful and striking dish!

The following recipe counts as 1 serving of vegetable.

Ingredients you will need for this recipe:

- Green onions, 45-degree bias sliced into 0.5-inch pieces (1 C.)

- Liquid amino acids (0.5 T.)

- Paprika (0.5 t.)

- Ground white peppercorns (0.5 t.)

- Sea salt (0.5 t.)

- Celery seed (0.125 t.)

- Cayenne powder or red pepper flakes (0.125 t.)

- Vegetable broth (2 C.)

How to prepare this recipe:

- Reserve a pinch of green onions on the side for garnish later.

- Preheat the saucepan over medium heat. Sauté the rest of the green onions for 2-3 minutes. Gradually, add spoonfuls of the water or broth as necessary to prevent from sticking.

- Add the spices and liquid amino acids. Sauté for another 1-2 minutes. Add the rest of the vegetable broth and bring to a boil.

- Lower the heat. For the next 20 minutes, keep at a simmer.

- Take it off the stovetop and transfer to a bowl to serve. Garnish with the remaining green onions.

Classic Egg Drop Soup

Egg drop soup is one of those items that you'll find on any Chinese-American restaurant menu. It's warm, comforting, and flavorful. This is a very easy and quick no-fuss soup! Additional spices can be added to alter the flavor of the soup based on your tastes; cinnamon, star anise, and other spices in the Chinese 5-spices family are some good choices. Feel free to vary the speed at which you pour in and whisk the eggs. If you whisk quickly, you'll get smaller bits of egg. If you pour in and whisk more slowly, you'll get longer, stringier egg elements.

The following recipe counts as 1 serving of protein and 1 serving of vegetable.

Ingredients you will need for this recipe:

- Chicken broth (2 C.)

- Liquid amino acids (1 T.)

- Green onions, thinly sliced (0.5 C.)

- Ground garlic (0.5 t.)

- Ground ginger (0.5 t.)

- Egg (1 whole) and egg whites (3, or approximately 0.5 C.)

- Ground black peppercorns and sea salt, to taste

How to prepare this recipe:

- Bring broth to a boil in a saucepan.

- Add all ingredients except for eggs, salt, and pepper.

- Whisk together the egg and egg whites. Slowly pour into the saucepan, while stirring soup continuously. Ribbons of eggs should appear in the soup.

- Turn off the stovetop, transfer to a bowl, and serve immediately. Add sea salt and ground black peppercorns to taste.

Chinese Chicken and Broccoli Soup

This is an all-star, one-pot soup requiring very little effort! The broccoli should be bright green and tender by the time the soup is finished. The notes of garlic, white pepper, and liquid amino acids give it a Chinese flair. White pepper rather than black pepper is more traditionally used in Chinese cuisine due to its fine texture and less intense flavor. However, feel free to substitute black pepper if your white pepper isn't available.

The following recipe counts as 1 serving of protein and 1 serving of vegetable.

Ingredients you will need for this recipe:

- Chicken, cubed (100 g)

- Broccoli, chopped (1 C.)

- Water (3 C.)

- Onion powder (1 t.)

- Ground garlic (1 t.)

- Ground cumin (1 t.)

- Ground white peppercorns (0.5 t.)

- Liquid amino acids (0.5 T.)

How to prepare this recipe:

- In a saucepan, cook the chicken until lightly browned. Add water in spoonfuls as necessary to prevent sticking.

- Add remaining ingredients to the saucepan. Allow soup to boil and then lower heat to keep at a simmer. Let keep at a simmer for 30 minutes, or until broccoli is tender.

- Turn off the stovetop, transfer to a bowl, and serve.

Banquet Imitation Shark Fin Soup

Shark fin soup is a fixture at Chinese banquets. It's typically brought out at very special events, such as weddings, New Year's celebrations, and birthdays. Shark fin soup made with authentic shark fins is rarely seen today due to exposure of the cruel techniques required to harvest the fins. This is a more compassionate version using zero-calorie konjac noodles as a replacement for shark fins. Crab meat and scallops give the soup that classic seafood flavor, while the konjac noodles provide texture and body to the soup.

The following recipe counts as 1 serving of protein and 1 serving of vegetable.

Ingredients you will need for this recipe:

- Konjac noodles (0.25 package)
- Vegetable broth (2-0.5 C.)
- Crab meat (2 t.)
- Scallops, dried (5 whole)
- Cabbage (1 C.)
- Sea salt (1 t.)
- Ground white peppercorns (1 t.)
- Liquid amino acids (0.5 T.)

How to prepare this recipe:

- Prepare the konjac noodles according to packaging. Set aside.
- Bring the broth to a boil and add the crab meat, scallops, and cabbage. Boil for 10 minutes.
- Add the konjac noodles, salt, white pepper, and liquid amino acids. Stir to combine well.
- Turn off the stovetop, transfer to a bowl, and serve.

Spinach Soup

This spinach soup is absolutely delicious with its notes of garlic and ginger. One of the really great things about spinach for the HCG diet is its relative lack of calories. You can eat many cups of spinach without feeling any guilt. Also, feel free to chop the spinach beforehand if you prefer smaller pieces mixed into the soup. Just note that the spinach will seem like a lot initially in its raw form. You'll be amazed at how drastically it'll shrink down once exposed to hot water!

The following recipe counts as 1 serving of vegetable.

Ingredients you will need for this recipe:

- Raw baby spinach (6 C.)

- Fresh minced garlic (a single clove)

- Fresh finely grated ginger (0.5 inches)

- Water or vegetable bouillon base (2-0.5 C.)

- Ground black peppercorns and sea salt, to taste

How to prepare this recipe:

- In a saucepan, sauté the garlic and ginger in 1 tablespoon of water or vegetable bouillon base.

- Add the remaining water or vegetable bouillon base. Allow it to come to a boil.

- Add the spinach and stir until it starts to wilt.

- Turn off the stovetop, transfer to a bowl, add the sea salt and ground black peppercorns to taste, and serve.

Simple Curry Chicken Soup

Curry is an ancient and traditional Asian spice, found in both eastern and southeastern Asian cuisines. It helps to warm the body, facilitating a faster metabolism. This curry chicken soup recipe is flavorful, but simple to make. In its base form, it is mild enough for kids and adults with a less spice-inclined palette to enjoy.

The following recipe counts as 1 serving of protein and 1 serving of vegetable.

Ingredients you will need for this recipe:

- Chicken (100 g)
- Onion, diced (1 C.)
- Fresh minced garlic (a single clove)
- Vegetable broth (2 C.)
- Curry powder, to taste (approximately 2 t.)
- Lemon juice (2 T.)
- Red pepper flakes (1 t.)
- Ground black peppercorns and sea salt, to taste

How to prepare this recipe:

- In a saucepan, sauté the chicken to a medium/high heat until opaque.
- Add the onion and garlic and stir until the chicken is browned and onion begins to turn translucent. Turn off the heat.
- Remove the chicken and shred it.
- Add the chicken, vegetable broth, curry powder, lemon juice, red pepper flakes, salt, and ground black peppercorns to the pan with the onion and garlic. Allow it to come to a boil.
- Turn off the stovetop, transfer to a bowl, and serve.

Ginger Beef Stew

This recipe turns the classic ginger beef dish into a soup, meaning that you can enjoy the classic flavors while getting that extra boost of hydration. Hearty steak pairs with delicious fresh onion to achieve that rich stew texture, without being as heavy and sleep-inducing as a traditional beef stew. Be sure to use lean steak in this, or else, you'll see bubbles of fat and oil melt off of the meat when you make the soup. It's definitely a good one to enjoy as a bowl of leftovers as well.

The following recipe counts as 1 serving of protein and 1 serving of vegetable. Optional: 1 Melba toast serving.

Ingredients you will need for this recipe:

- Lean steak, cut into chunks (100 g)
- Ground ginger (1 t.)
- Onion powder (1 t.)
- Ground black peppercorns and sea salt, to taste
- Onion, chopped (1 C.)
- Fresh minced garlic (2 cloves)
- Bay leaf (1)
- Beef broth (2 C.)
- Melba toast (1 piece) (optional)

How to prepare this recipe:

- Season the steak with ginger, onion powder, sea salt, and ground black peppercorns.
- Add the steak, chopped onion, and garlic to a saucepan. Sauté on med-high heat until the steak is browned. Add spoonfuls of the beef broth, if necessary, to avoid sticking.

- Add the bay leaf and beef broth. Allow it to come to a boil.

- Lower the heat to low-medium and keep at a simmer for 45 minutes. If necessary, add the water to its preferred consistency.

- Turn off the stovetop, transfer to a bowl, and take out bay leaf.

- Serve with Melba toast, if you desire.

Cabbage and Beef Soup

This cabbage and beef soup is light but will still fill you up! The whole cup of cabbage helps it feel substantial. The dried cilantro is optional but makes for a nice visual when sprinkled on top immediately before serving.

The following recipe counts as 1 serving of protein and 1 serving of vegetable.

Ingredients you will need for this recipe for this recipe:

- Lean steak, chopped into 1-inch pieces (100 g)
- Onion powder (1 t.)
- Ground garlic (1 t.)
- Ginger powder (0.5 t.)
- Ground black peppercorns and sea salt, to taste
- Cabbage, chopped (1 C.)
- Beef broth (2 C.)
- Liquid amino acids (1 t.)
- Dried cilantro (1 t.) (optional)

How to prepare this recipe:

- Season the steak with the onion powder, garlic powder, ginger, salt, and pepper.
- In a saucepan, sauté until lightly browned. Add spoonfuls of the beef broth as necessary to prevent sticking.
- Add the cabbage to the saucepan. Sauté for a couple minutes until cabbage begins to turn translucent.
- Add the beef broth, liquid amino acids, and dried cilantro, if using. Allow it to come to a boil.
- Lower the heat and keep at a simmer for 30 minutes. Turn off the stovetop, transfer to a bowl, and serve.

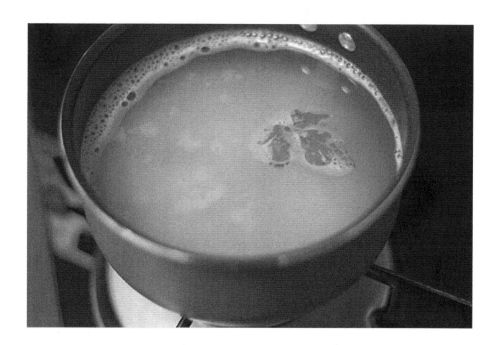

Easy Chicken Broth

What home chef's recipe book would be complete without a broth recipe? Homemade broth eliminates the possibility of finding high amounts of salt, sugar, and added chemicals in your broth, which is typical of many different store-bought varieties. This is meant to be a base recipe for your creativity. Feel free to add in whichever spices you prefer. With these general directions, you can also make a fantastic beef or vegetable broth, depending on what dish you plan on using the broth for. It can be really handy to have the broth ready for whenever you need it, so we suggest making a big batch beforehand (double or triple the recipe) and freezing it for later.

Ingredients you will need for this recipe:

- Water (3 C.)

- Chicken (100 g)

- Ground garlic, optional, to taste

- Onion powder, optional, to taste

- Rosemary, optional, to taste

- Thyme, optional, to taste

- Basil, optional, to taste

- Bay leaf, optional, to taste

- White or black pepper, optional, to taste

- Sea salt, optional, to taste

How to prepare this recipe:

- In a saucepan, allow the water to boil.

- Add the chicken and seasonings as desired. Boil for at least 30 minutes.

- Remove the chicken and save for a separate recipe.

- Strain out the seasonings, if you desire. Let the broth cool to the touch and then skim the floating fat off the surface if visible.

- Refrigerate or freeze the broth, if not using immediately.

Asparagus and Chicken Salad With Ginger Dressing

This is a delicious and filling salad. The ginger dressing brings a hint of Asian flair to the salad. The asparagus and chicken provide great texture, and sprigs of herbs add a delightful freshness.

The following recipe counts as 1 serving of protein and 1 serving of vegetable.

Ingredients you will need for this recipe:

For the dressing:

- Onion powder (0.5 T.)

- Vinegar (apple cider) (1 T.)

- Stevia (0.5 T.)

- Mustard powder (0.25 tbsp.)

- Ground black peppercorns and sea salt, to taste

- Cayenne powder (a pinch)

- Fresh finely grated ginger (0.25-inch piece)

- Fresh minced garlic (a single clove)

For the salad:

- Lean chicken, thinly sliced (100 g)

- Asparagus (5 stalks)

- Ground black peppercorns and sea salt, to taste

- Lime (0.5 lime)

- Fresh herbs, optional, to taste

How to prepare this recipe:

- To make the dressing, mix together in a small bowl the onion powder, vinegar, Stevia, mustard powder, salt, pepper, cayenne powder, ginger, and garlic. Stir well to combine and refrigerate while making asparagus.

- Heat a wok (or sauté pan) on medium/high heat. Add the chicken and then the water in spoonfuls as necessary to prevent from sticking. Stir occasionally until chicken is browned. Use a meat thermometer if necessary to check the internal temperature of chicken (at least 165 degrees Fahrenheit).

- Take the chicken out of the pan and set aside.

- Cut off the tough end (about 0.5–1 inch) of each asparagus spear and then slice each spear into 2-inch pieces. Slice thicker asparagus pieces in half lengthwise as necessary so that all pieces are bite-sized and the same size approximately.

- Bring a pot of water to boil.

- Place the asparagus into the boiling water. Cook for a couple minutes or until bright green and just tender. Drain and then rinse. Dry with either paper towels or a tea towel.

- To prepare the salad, add the asparagus to a bowl and add the salt and ground black peppercorns if desired. Add half of the vinaigrette and thoroughly toss to fully coat the asparagus.

- Arrange the asparagus on the plate. Shred the chicken or leave as strips and place over the asparagus. Drizzle the remaining vinaigrette on top.

- Serve immediately.

Simple Chinese Cucumber Salad

Cucumbers are a very popular snack in China! During the summer, people can be seen just eating cucumbers whole. This salad takes inspiration from that and is perfect for a light, refreshing lunch.

The following recipe counts as 1 serving of vegetable.

Ingredients you will need for this recipe:

- Vinegar (apple cider) (4 T.)

- Ground garlic (0.5 t.)

- Ground ginger (0.25 t.)

- Ground white peppercorns (0.25 t.)

- Sea salt (0.25 t.)

- Stevia, to taste

- Cucumber, sliced into bite-sized chunks (1 whole cucumber)

How to prepare this recipe:

- Take a small bowl and combine the vinegar, garlic powder, ground ginger, white pepper, salt, and stevia.

- Add the cucumber pieces to a bowl. Pour the sauce mixture over cucumbers and mix well.

- Marinate for an hour in the refrigerator before serving.

Chapter 4

Vegetable Sides

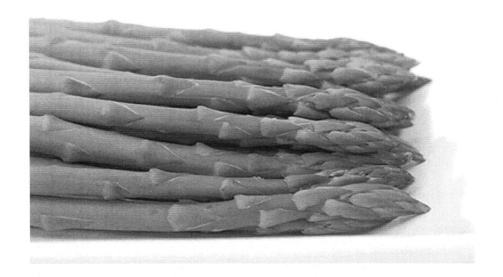

Quick and Simple Orange Asparagus

Orange juice and orange zest add a very fresh feeling to this asparagus dish! As this dish is prepared in the oven, you won't have to spend time hovering over your stovetop. Enjoy with more orange zest sprinkled on top, if desired.

The following recipe counts as 1 vegetable and 0.5 fruit serving.

Ingredients you will need for this recipe:

- Asparagus (5 stalks)

- Orange zest (from 1 orange)

- Orange juice (0.5 orange)

- Ground black peppercorns and sea salt, to taste

How to prepare this recipe:

- Preheat the oven to 375 degrees Fahrenheit.

- Add the asparagus to a baking dish. Sprinkle the remaining ingredients on top.

- Cook for 5 to 10 minutes or until a fork can pierce the asparagus stems.

- Serve immediately.

Sweet and Sour Cabbage Slaw

This recipe takes the classic Chinese-American sweet and sour flavors and pairs it with a delicious and fresh cabbage slaw. The cabbage retains its satisfying crunch, and the texture of the leaves really hold on well to the sweet and sour sauce. Enjoy with a sprinkle of black pepper on top.

The following recipe counts as 1 serving of vegetable.

Ingredients you will need for this recipe:

- Vinegar (apple cider) (2 T., or to taste)

- Liquid amino acids (0.5 t.)

- Stevia, to taste

- Ground black peppercorns and sea salt, to taste

- Cabbage, chopped thinly (1 C.)

How to prepare this recipe:

- Take a small bowl and combine the vinegar, liquid amino acids, stevia, salt, and freshly ground pepper.

- Add the cabbage to a bowl and drizzle the vinegar mixture over. Stir well to combine.

- Refrigerate to chill to a preferred temperature and then serve immediately.

General Tso's Cauliflower

Who knew cauliflower paired so well with the spice of a General Tso's sauce? The texture of the cauliflower mimics that of a breaded piece of chicken or beef. Feel free to amp up the spice levels if you are ready for it!

The following recipe counts as 1 serving of vegetable.

Ingredients you will need for this recipe:

For the sauce:

- Vinegar (apple cider) (1 T.)

- Liquid amino acids (1-0.5 T.)

- Vegetable broth or water (0.125 C.)

- Stevia (1 packet)

For the cauliflower:

- Cauliflower (2 C.)

- Sea salt (1 t.)

- Fresh finely grated ginger (0.5 T.)

- Fresh minced garlic (a single clove)

- Dried Chinese red chilies (5 whole) or red pepper flakes (0.5 T., or to taste)

- Green onions, 45-degree bias sliced into 0.5-inch pieces (1 C.)

How to prepare this recipe:

- Take a small bowl and mix together the ingredients listed for the sauce. Set aside.

- Heat a large sauté pan or wok to a medium/high heat. Add the cauliflower and salt and then add water in spoonfuls as necessary to prevent from sticking. Stir occasionally until cauliflower is tender.

- Remove the cauliflower and set aside.

- Reduce the heat to medium and add the garlic, ginger, and red chilies (or red pepper flakes). Add a spoonful of water. Stir for 30 seconds or when you start to smell the spices.

- Add the cauliflower, sauce mixture, and green onions to the sauté pan. Stir until combined.

- Turn off the stovetop, transfer to a bowl, and serve.

Summertime Chinese Smashed Cucumbers With Garlic

Smashed cucumbers are a classic Chinese dish. Garlic and red pepper flakes add a refreshing kick. It's a summertime staple but delicious all year round.

The following recipe counts as 1 serving of vegetable.

Ingredients you will need for this recipe:

- Cucumber, thin-skinned variety, such as English/Persian (1 whole cucumber)

- Sea salt (0.25 t., plus a dash for cucumbers)

- Stevia (0.5 t., plus a dash for cucumbers)

- Vinegar (apple cider) (1 t.)

- Liquid amino acids (0.5 t.)

- Fresh minced garlic (a single clove)

- Red pepper flakes, to taste

How to prepare this recipe:

- Wash and dry the cucumber. Cut into 3 sections and then cut each section in half lengthwise.

- Lay down a single chunk of cucumber on a hard, flat surface. Place the flat side of a large cutting knife against the cucumber and smash down lightly repeatedly with your hand (similar to how you might smash a garlic clove). This is a classic Chinese technique. Continue until the cucumber has cracked, with the skin and flesh looking smashed.

- Cut the smashed cucumbers into small, bite-sized pieces. Remove the cucumber seeds.

33

- Place cucumber pieces into a strainer and mix with a dash of salt and sugar. If possible, place something over the cucumbers to act as a weight, such as a bag of ice.

- Let the cucumbers drain for approximately half an hour on the counter or in the refrigerator (up to 4 hours maximum).

- In the meantime, prepare the sauce. Take a small bowl and combine the salt, stevia, and vinegar. Stir until combined well and then add the liquid amino acids.

- When ready to serve the cucumbers, shake the strainer to rid cucumbers of extra liquid. Lightly dry with a paper towel if excessively wet.

- Transfer to a bowl. Mix the cucumbers with sauce and the remaining ingredients.

- Serve immediately.

Garlic Baby Spinach

Who doesn't love a big batch of garlicky greens? Feel free to bump up the spinach or garlic in this recipe. This makes a particularly fantastic side to the General Tso's chicken recipe featured later in this book.

The following recipe counts as 1 serving of vegetable.

Ingredients you will need for this recipe:

- Raw baby spinach (6 C.)

- Fresh minced garlic (a single clove)

- Water or vegetable bouillon base (6 T.)

How to prepare this recipe:

- In a big saucepan or sauté pan, sauté the garlic in a spoonful of water or vegetable bouillon base.

- Add the remaining water or vegetable bouillon base and spinach.

- Stir until it starts to wilt. Turn off the stovetop, transfer to a bowl, and serve.

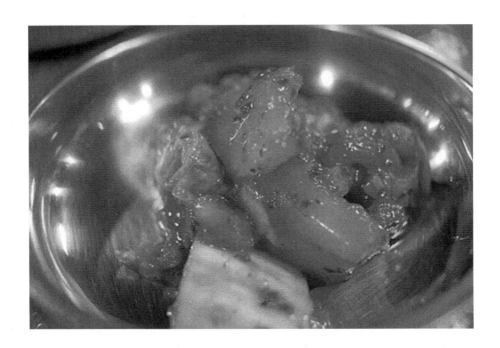

Restaurant Pickled Cabbage

Pickled cabbage is a common appetizer at Chinese restaurants. Reminiscent of the Korean dish kimchi, the cabbage in this recipe retains a delicious vinegary taste and soft bite. Make a big batch and enjoy a small portion every day for the rest of the week.

The following recipe counts as 1 serving of vegetable.

Ingredients you will need for this recipe:

- Cabbage (0.5 cabbage)
- Sea salt (2 T.)
- Water (0.5 C.)
- Stevia (0.25 C.)
- Red pepper flakes (0.25 t. or more, to taste)
- Vinegar (apple cider) (0.25 C.)
- Garlic, minced (a single clove)

How to prepare this recipe:

- In a big mixing bowl, rip the cabbage by hand into fairly large pieces, approximately 3-inch square. They may seem large now, but they will shrink after pickling.

- Pour in the salt. Using your hands, mix and thoroughly and evenly distribute the salt among the cabbage shreds. Top the cabbage with some sort of clean, wrapped heavy object. Let it marinate for between 45 minutes and an hour in the refrigerator. This will allow the cabbage to rid itself of excess liquid, and the cabbage will be extra crunchy. However, refrain from marinating for too long or the cabbage will taste too salty. Check at 45 minutes to test salt levels.

- In a separate saucepan, combine water, stevia, and red pepper flakes. Bring to boil and turn off the heat. Stir in the vinegar and another dash of salt. Let the liquid cool to room temperature. With a spoon, taste the liquid and determine if you like the level of sweet and sour. Adjust accordingly.

- Once the cabbage has marinated appropriately, wash them to fully get rid of the salt. This may take 2 to 3 rinses. Squeeze out any extra liquid. Wrap with a clean tea towel or paper towels if necessary to make them just slightly damp to the touch.

- Place the cabbage in a bowl. Add the garlic to the cabbage.

- Pour the vinegar and water mixture over the cabbage and stir gently to combine.

- Wrap with plastic wrap or cover with lid. Move to the refrigerator for at least one day before serving chilled. Leftovers should be stored in the pickling juice until consumed.

Grilled Onion and Garlic Cabbage Wedges

This is a hearty and delicious grilled dish! The cabbage has a fantastic crunch, and the wedge form makes it feel very substantial. It's a great summertime side!

The following recipe counts as 1 serving of vegetable.

Ingredients you will need for this recipe:

- Cabbage, wedged (0.5 cabbage)

- Ground garlic (1 t.)

- Onion powder (1 t.)

- Ground black peppercorns and sea salt, to taste

How to prepare this recipe:

- Preheat the oven to 450 degrees Fahrenheit.

- Wrap the cabbage wedges in an aluminum foil.

- Pour a couple of spoonfuls of water for steaming over the cabbage.

- Sprinkle the remaining ingredients onto the cabbage.

- Close the aluminum foil and grill for approximately 20 to 25 minutes or until tender.

Garlic Lemon Chard

Chard is a powerhouse of vitamins and minerals; chard is packed with Vitamins A, C, and K. Enjoy rainbow Swiss chard for a truly beautiful and visual dish that everyone will love.

The following recipe counts as 1 serving of vegetable.

Ingredients you will need for this recipe:

- Fresh minced garlic (2 cloves)

- Swiss chard (0.5 bunch)

- Lemon juice (2 T.)

- Ground black peppercorns and sea salt, to taste

How to prepare this recipe:

- In a sauté pan, brown the garlic for a couple minutes until fragrant. Add water as necessary to prevent sticking.

- Add the Swiss chard, lemon juice, salt, and pepper. Cook until the chard wilts.

- Turn off the stovetop, transfer to a bowl, and serve immediately.

Steamed Mustard Cabbage

Classic steamed cabbage gets a boost of flavor with tangy lemon juice and mustard! Enjoy paired with orange chicken to complement the citrus notes.

The following recipe counts as 1 serving of vegetable.

Ingredients you will need for this recipe:

- Water (0.25 C.)

- Cabbage, chopped into thin slices (0.5 cabbage)

- Lemon juice (0.5 lemons)

- Spicy mustard (0.5 t.)

- Ground black peppercorns and sea salt, to taste

How to prepare this recipe:

- In a saucepan, add the water and bring to a boil.

- Add the cabbage to the saucepan, lower the heat, and steam for 5 to 10 minutes or until tender.

- Take a small bowl and stir together the mustard and the juice of a lemon.

- Drain the cabbage and mix it with the lemon/mustard mixture.

- Add the sea salt and ground black peppercorns on top and serve immediately.

Caramelized Onions

Caramelized onions are found in many different cuisines, so this is a recipe you can keep on hand for future dishes as well! The natural sweetness and caramelization can satisfy any sugar craving with the benefit of added Vitamin C and fiber.

The following recipe counts as 1 serving of vegetable.

Ingredients you will need for this recipe:

- Onion, chopped into thin slices (1 whole)

- Vegetable broth or water (0.25 C.)

- Thyme (0.25 t.) (optional)

- Ground black peppercorns and sea salt, to taste

How to prepare this recipe:

- Heat a large sauté pan on medium/high.

- Place the onion slices into the pan and add a dash of salt. Let it sit for 5 minutes without moving around. This will allow the onions to caramelize. Lower the heat if the onions start to burn or smoke.

- Stir the onions, ensuring that the onions have started to brown and caramelize. Flip the onions to allow all sides to brown. Use a wooden spoon to start scraping the bottom and sides of the pan down. Add a few spoonfuls of vegetable broth or water to assist in the deglazing process.

- When the onions are fully translucent, add the rest of the vegetable broth or water as well as the other spices, salt, and pepper. Once again, use the wooden spoon to scrape the bottom and sides of the pan down and to fully deglaze the pan.

- Continue until the onions are caramelized to its preferred tenderness, and liquid has evaporated.

- Turn off the stovetop, transfer to a bowl, and serve immediately.

Chapter 5

Main Courses

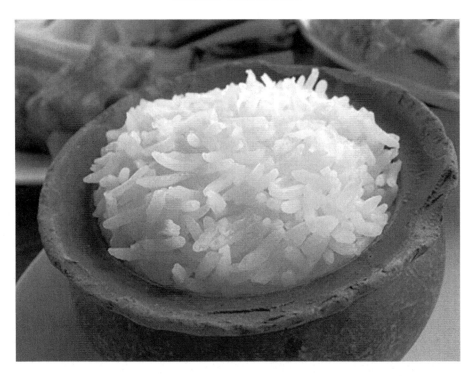

HCG-Friendly Konjac Rice

Konjac rice is an amazing grain-free, low-carb, zero-calorie rice made from water and konjac plant fiber. It is largely accepted by dieters as being HCG-friendly, but it's up to each person to determine whether they're comfortable adding them to their plan. In addition to konjac rice, konjac is also used to make various types of noodles! You can have a big, heaping bowl of Chinese chow fun, ho fun, chow mein, or lo mein and still stick with your diet protocol. Many brands exist, so check the ingredients before you purchase to make sure it doesn't have any extra ingredients. Konjac rice allows you to have a heaping scoop of warm rice, a staple of every Chinese-American dish!

Ingredients you will need for this recipe:

- Konjac rice (0.5 C.)

- Water (1 C.)

Different brands may require different preparations. Refer to the rice packaging for exact cooking times.

How to prepare this recipe:

- Rinse thoroughly with water for a minute.

- Allow the water to boil.

- Add the rice and boil for a minute.

- Dry the rice either by sandwiching between paper towels or by adding it to a pan over the heat until dry.

- Serve immediately.

Simple Egg Fried Rice

Fried rice is a classic Chinese restaurant dish! This is especially quick to whip up if you have some leftover Konjac rice on hand. Fresh chopped onion and garlic give this dish fantastic flavor, and the egg makes it filling.

The following recipe counts as 1 serving of protein and 1 serving of vegetable.

Ingredients you will need for this recipe:

- Konjac rice (0.5 C.)

- Water (1 C.)

- Onion, chopped finely (0.5 onion)

- Garlic, minced (2 cloves)

- Egg (1 whole) and egg whites (3, or approximately 0.5 C.)

- Liquid Amino Acids (2 T.)

- Ground black peppercorns and sea salt, to taste

Different brands of rice may require different preparations. Refer to the rice packaging for exact cooking times.

How to prepare this recipe:

- Rinse the konjac rice thoroughly with water for a minute.

- Allow the water to boil.

- Add the rice and boil for a minute.

- Dry the rice either by sandwiching between paper towels or by adding it to a pan over the heat until dry.

- Separately, heat a sauté pan or wok over medium heat. Sauté the onions and garlic until fragrant. Add spoonfuls of water as necessary to prevent from sticking.

- Whisk together egg and egg whites and add to sauté pan. Cook for a couple minutes, scrambling the egg as it cooks.

- Stir in the rice, liquid amino acids, salt, and ground black peppercorns. Mix gently.

- Turn off the stovetop, transfer to a bowl, and serve immediately.

General Tso's Chicken

General Tso's chicken is a mainstay at all Chinese-American restaurants. The combination of the sweet, tangy, and spice make this an absolutely delectable dish. In this recipe, scallions are also cut on the bias, adding an element of visual interest.

The following recipe counts as 1 serving of protein.

Ingredients you will need for this recipe:

For the sauce:

- Vinegar (apple cider) (1 T.)

- Liquid amino acids (1 0.5 T.)

- Vegetable broth or water (0.125 C.)

- Stevia (1 packet)

For the chicken:

- Lean chicken, cut into 1-inch pieces (100 g)

- Sea salt (a pinch)

- Fresh finely grated ginger (0.5 T.)

- Fresh minced garlic (a single clove)

- Dried Chinese red chilies (5 whole) or red pepper flakes (0.5 T. or to taste)

- Green onions, 45-degree bias sliced into 0.5-inch pieces (1 C.)

How to prepare this recipe:

- Take a small bowl and mix together the ingredients listed for the sauce. Set aside.

- Heat a large sauté pan or wok to a medium/high heat. Add the chicken and salt and then add the water in spoonfuls as necessary to prevent from sticking. Stir occasionally until the chicken is browned. Use a meat thermometer if necessary to check the internal temperature of the chicken (at least 165 degrees Fahrenheit).

- Take the chicken out of the pan and set aside.

- Reduce the heat to medium and add the garlic, ginger, and red chilies (or red pepper flakes). Add a spoonful of water. Stir for 30 seconds or when you start to smell the spices.

- Add the chicken, sauce mixture, and green onions to the sauté pan. Stir until combined.

- Turn off the stovetop, transfer to a bowl, and serve.

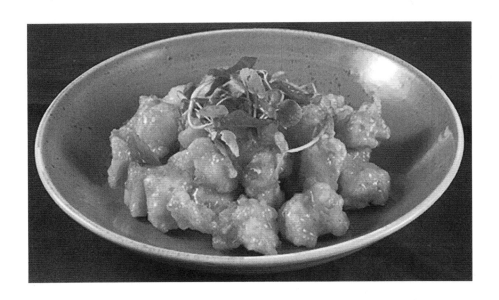

Easy Orange Chicken

Orange chicken is found on every Chinese-American restaurant menu, and this is a simple and quick version that you can easily make at home! The color is absolutely gorgeous thanks to the orange zest. Enjoy with a big bowl of fresh konjac rice.

The following recipe counts as 1 serving of protein and 1 serving of fruit.

Ingredients you will need for this recipe:

- Lean chicken, cut into bite-sized chunks (100 g)

- Orange zest (1 orange)

- Orange juice (1 orange)

- Vegetable broth (0.5 C.)

- Onion, diced into small pieces (2 t.)

- Ginger, grated (2 t.)

- Vinegar (apple cider) (2 T.)

- Ground garlic (0.25 t.)

- Ground black peppercorns and sea salt, to taste

- Stevia, to taste

How to prepare this recipe:

- Heat a sauté pan or wok to a medium/high heat.

- Add all ingredients to the sauté pan. Cook until the chicken is thoroughly cooked, and the liquid has been reduced to preferred consistency. Use a meat thermometer if necessary to check the internal temperature of the chicken (at least 165 degrees Fahrenheit).

- Serve immediately.

Ginger Orange Chicken Wraps

Fresh, delicious ginger orange wraps make a great lunch or dinner. Take care to use really large lettuce leaves to make sure you can wrap the chicken properly without any escapees.

The following recipe counts as 1 serving of protein and 1 serving of vegetable. Optional: 1 Melba toast serving.

Ingredients you will need for this recipe:

- Lean chicken, cubed into bite-sized pieces (100 g)

- Lettuce (2 large leaves)

- Fresh minced garlic (2 cloves)

- Onion, minced (2 t.)

- Ground ginger (0.25 t.)

- Ground black peppercorns and sea salt, to taste

- Orange, peeled and chopped into bite-sized pieces (1 orange)

- Orange zest (1 orange)

- Lemon juice (0.5 lemon)

- Melba toast (1 piece) (optional)

How to prepare this recipe:

- Heat a large sauté pan to a medium/high heat. Add the chicken. Add the water in spoonfuls as necessary to prevent from sticking. Add the garlic, onion, ginger, salt, and pepper. Stir occasionally until the chicken is browned. Use a meat thermometer if necessary to check the internal temperature of the chicken (at least 165 degrees Fahrenheit).

- Turn off the stovetop and transfer to a bowl.

- Spread out the lettuce leaves on a plate. Add the chicken to the center of the lettuce. Add the orange pieces, orange zest, and additional sea salt and ground black peppercorns, if you desire. Add the lemon juice to each wrap. Wrap the lettuce leaves over into hand-sized wraps.

- Serve with Melba toast, if you desire.

Dim Sum Chicken Meatballs

Dim sum is a characteristically Chinese meal event. Small dishes are pushed around on carts and shared among families, so everyone gets to try a bunch of different bite-sized treats! These meatballs are often found on the dim sum carts garnished with cilantro and dipped in soy sauce. This recipe is an HCG-friendly version! Feel free to make a big batch and freeze meatballs before cooking to enjoy later without the hassle of preparation.

The following recipe counts as 1 serving of protein and 1 serving of vegetable.

Ingredients you will need for this recipe:

- Lean ground chicken (100 g)

- Melba toast smashed into small crumbs (1 piece)

- Ground garlic (0.25 t.)

- Onion powder (0.25 t.)

- Ground ginger (0.25 t.)

- Ground white peppercorns (0.25 t.)

- Liquid amino acids (2 t.)

- Dried cilantro (0.25 t.)

- Cabbage, chopped into thin slices (1 C.)

How to prepare this recipe:

- In a big bowl, combine the ground chicken, Melba toast, garlic powder, onion powder, ground ginger, white pepper, liquid amino acids, and cilantro. Use a spoon or fork and mash to combine well.

- Using a spoon and your hands, grab pieces of the chicken mixture, rolling the mixture to create meatballs approximately 1 0.5-inch to 2-inch wide. Wash hands thoroughly.

- Heat a large sauté pan over medium heat. Arrange the meatballs inside the pan, and add a few spoonfuls of water to prevent from sticking. Place lid on top.

- After a couple minutes, check under the lid. If the water is close to evaporating, add a few more spoonfuls of water, enough to deglaze the bottom of the pan. Stir the meatballs and replace the lid on top. Continue the process until the meatballs are cooked through. Use a meat thermometer if necessary to check the internal temperature of the chicken (at least 165 degrees Fahrenheit).

- Remove the lid and stir the meatballs to brown lightly on the exterior. Turn the heat up to high if necessary to facilitate browning. Turn off the stovetop, transfer to a bowl, and set aside.

- Deglaze the sauté pan with water once more. Add the cabbage and cook to desired tenderness and consistency.

- Serve the chicken meatballs with cabbage immediately.

Classic Chicken Stir-Fry

What Chinese cookbook would be complete without a stir-fry recipe? This recipe allows for so many different variations, and the biggest benefit is how quick it is. Using a very hot wok for pan will allow for fast cooking and a speedy dinner on the table.

The following recipe counts as 1 serving of protein and 1 serving of vegetable.

Ingredients you will need for this recipe:

For the sauce:

- Liquid amino acids (0.5 T.)

- Lime juice (0.25 T.)

- Water (0.5 T.)

For the chicken:

- Lean chicken, sliced into thin strips (100 g)

- Fresh minced garlic (0.5 t.)

- Ginger, grated (0.5 t.)

- Broccoli, roughly chopped into small florets and stems (1 C.)

- Ground black peppercorns and sea salt, to taste

How to prepare this recipe:

- Combine the sauce ingredients in a small bowl. Set aside.

- Heat a large sauté pan or wok to a medium/high heat. Add the chicken and salt and then add the water in spoonfuls as necessary to prevent from sticking. Stir occasionally until the chicken is browned. Use a meat thermometer if necessary to check the internal temperature of the chicken (at least 165 degrees Fahrenheit).

- Take the chicken out of the pan and set aside.

- Reduce the heat to medium and add the garlic and ginger. Add a spoonful of water. Stir for 30 seconds or when you start to smell the spices. Add the broccoli and cook until tender (about 5 minutes). Add the water as necessary.

- Add the chicken and liquid amino sauce mixture to the sauté pan. Stir until combined.

- Turn off the stovetop, transfer to a bowl, and serve.

Simple Garlic Chicken

Roasting this chicken in the oven means less work for you! This recipe has a really fantastic garlic and lemon flavor. Feel free to boost the number of garlic cloves used.

The following recipe counts as 1 serving of protein and 1 serving of vegetable.

Ingredients you will need for this recipe:

- Onion, chopped into slices (0.5 C.)

- Garlic, unpeeled and roughly chopped into large pieces (4 cloves or to taste)

- Lean chicken (100 g)

- Lemon juice (0.5 lemon)

- Ground black peppercorns and sea salt, to taste

How to prepare this recipe:

- Preheat the oven to 350 degrees.

- Heat a sauté pan over medium heat.

- Add the onion and stir constantly until nearly translucent.

- Remove the onions and transfer to a glass baking dish. Add the chicken, placing on top of the onions. Add the lemon juice on top and sprinkle with sea salt and ground black peppercorns, if you desire. Put the garlic around and on top of the chicken. Wrap with aluminum foil, being sure to seal well.

- Place in the oven on middle rack and roast for approximately 30 to 45 minutes or until the chicken's internal temperature reaches 165 degrees Fahrenheit.

Low-Fat Sweet and Sour Chicken

This is a great take on Chinese-American sweet and sour chicken, with a lot of fewer calories and fat than the restaurant version. Thinly sliced onion provides sweetness and a visual contrast to the chicken. Enjoy with a side of konjac rice.

The following recipe counts as 1 serving of protein, 1 serving of vegetable, and 1 serving of fruit.

Ingredients you will need for this recipe:

- Lean chicken, cut into bite-sized cubes (100 g)
- Water (1 C.)
- Lemon (0.5 lemon)
- Orange (0.5 orange)
- Onion, cut into thin slices (1 onion)
- Fresh minced garlic (a single clove)
- Liquid Aminos (3 T.)
- Ground ginger (0.25 t.)
- Cayenne powder, to taste
- Ground black peppercorns and sea salt, to taste

How to prepare this recipe:

- Heat a large sauté pan to a medium/high heat. Add the chicken. Add the water in spoonfuls as necessary to prevent from sticking. Stir occasionally until the chicken is browned. Use a meat thermometer if necessary to check the internal temperature of the chicken (at least 165 degrees Fahrenheit).
- Take the chicken out of the pan and set aside.

- In a saucepan, bring the water to a boil.

- Add the lemon and orange, including the rind. Boil until the citrus pulp separates from the rind, coming out of the center.

- Remove the citrus rinds from the saucepan. If excess pulp clings to the rinds, scrape out the leftover pulp. Discard the rinds.

- Add the onion slices, garlic, liquid amino acids, ginger, cayenne, salt, and pepper. Reduce the liquid by about half, stirring once in a while.

- Reduce the heat to medium and add the chicken to the sauce. Stir until combined.

- Turn off the stovetop, transfer to a bowl, and serve immediately.

Beef Egg Roll Bowl

Now, you can enjoy a classic egg roll without the oil and fat of the crispy skin! These flavors are spot on similar to that of an egg roll. Enjoy with extra ginger, onion, or garlic, if desired.

The following recipe counts as 1 serving of protein and 1 serving of vegetable.

Ingredients you will need for this recipe:

- Lean ground beef (100 g)

- Onion powder (0.5 t.)

- Ground garlic (0.5 t.)

- Ginger powder (0.5 t.)

- Cabbage, chopped (1 0.5 C.)

- Liquid Aminos (1 T.)

- Water (1 T.)

- Stevia (1 packet)

- Ground black peppercorns and sea salt, to taste

How to prepare this recipe:

- In a sauté pan or wok, brown the ground beef with the spices until fragrant and browned. Add the water in spoonfuls as necessary to prevent from sticking.

- Add the cabbage, liquid amino acids, stevia, and water. Place a lid on top and then steam for approximately 10 minutes or until cabbage reaches desired softness.

- Turn off the stovetop, transfer to a bowl, add the sea salt and ground black peppercorns to taste, and serve.

Beef Konjac Chow Fun Noodles

Chow fun noodles are a staple among Chinese-American diners. The chewy, soy sauce-soaked flavor makes these noodles addictive, and the konjac noodles and liquid amino acids make them guilt-free! Take care to be careful with the noodles to avoid sticking and breakage.

The following recipe counts as 1 serving of protein and 1 serving of vegetable.

Ingredients you will need for this recipe:

- Lean steak, thinly sliced (100 g)

- Beef stock or water (4 T.)

- Fresh minced garlic (2 cloves)

- Onion, chopped into small pieces (1 C.)

- Onion powder (1 t.)

- Fresh finely grated ginger (1-inch piece)

- Konjac noodles (1 serving)

- Liquid amino acids (2 T.)

- Ground black peppercorns and sea salt, to taste

How to prepare this recipe:

- In a big saucepan or sauté pan, add the beef until very lightly browned. Add spoonfuls of the beef stock or water if necessary to prevent from sticking.

- Add the remaining beef stock or water, fresh minced garlic, onion, onion powder, and ginger and cook until the onion is tender and the beef is fully browned. Lower the heat to low.

- In a separate pot, prepare the konjac noodles according to packaging.

- Dry the konjac noodles by patting lightly with paper towels. Add the konjac noodles to the beef sauté pan and drizzle the liquid amino acids over everything. Stir gently to combine.

- Turn off the stovetop, transfer to a bowl, and serve immediately. Season with salt and ground black peppercorns as desired.

Ginger Beef and Onions

The different spices in this recipe create a wealth of flavors! Add extra red pepper flakes, if you're looking for an extra kick. Enjoy with a side of Konjac rice.

The following recipe counts as 1 serving of protein and 1 serving of vegetable.

Ingredients you will need for this recipe:

- Lean steak, thinly sliced (100 g)
- Beef stock or water (4 T.)
- Onion, cut into thin slices (1 onion)
- Liquid amino acids (1 0.5 T.)
- Fresh minced garlic (2 cloves)
- Ginger, grated (1-inch piece)
- Onion powder (1 t.)
- Ground cumin (0.125 t.)
- Red pepper flakes (0.125 t.)
- Ground black peppercorns and sea salt, to taste

How to prepare this recipe:

- In a big saucepan or sauté pan or wok, add the steak until very lightly browned. Add spoonfuls of the beef stock or water if necessary to prevent from sticking.
- Add the remaining ingredients to the pan and cook until the onion is tender and translucent and the beef is fully browned. Use a meat thermometer if necessary to check the internal temperature of the beef (at least 165-170 degrees Fahrenheit).
- Turn off the stovetop, transfer to a bowl, and serve immediately.

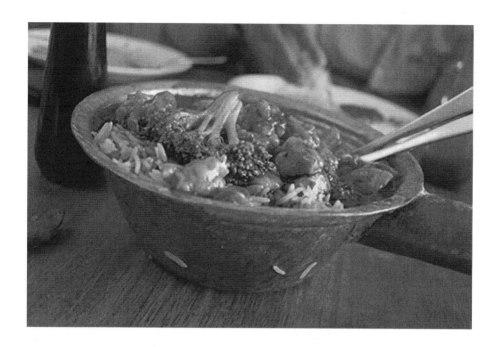

Healthy Beef and Broccoli

This is a healthy and easy take on classic beef and broccoli. Chopping your broccoli pieces will allow for quicker cooking. Note that the dried cilantro is optional.

The following recipe counts as 1 serving of protein and 1 serving of vegetable.

Ingredients you will need for this recipe:

- Lean steak, thinly sliced (100 g)

- Beef stock or water (4 T.)

- Broccoli, chopped into small pieces (1 C.)

- Liquid amino acids (1-0.5 T.)

- Fresh minced garlic (2 cloves)

- Onion powder (1 t.)

- Ground ginger (0.25 t.)

- Dried cilantro (0.5 t.) (optional)

How to prepare this recipe:

- In a big saucepan or sauté pan or wok, add the beef until very lightly browned. Add spoonfuls of the beef stock or water if necessary to prevent from sticking.

- Add the remaining ingredients to the pan and cook until the broccoli is tender and the beef is fully browned. Use a meat thermometer if necessary to check the internal temperature of the beef (at least 165-170 degrees Fahrenheit).

- Turn off the stovetop, transfer to a bowl, and serve immediately.

Ginger Steak and Tomato Skewers

These skewers are visually striking, with the array of steak and colorful tomatoes! Opt for heirloom cherry tomatoes at the grocery store, and you'll get a rainbow of yellow, orange, and red.

The following recipe counts as 1 serving of protein and 1 serving of vegetable.

Ingredients you will need for this recipe:

- Lemon juice (2 T.)

- Fresh finely grated ginger (2 t.)

- Fresh minced garlic (a single clove)

- Stevia, to taste

- Ground black peppercorns and sea salt, to taste

- Lean steak, cubed (100 g)

- Cherry tomatoes (4-5)

How to prepare this recipe:

- In a bowl, combine the lemon juice, ginger, garlic, stevia, salt, and pepper.

- Add the cubed steak. Cover with plastic wrap and marinate for at least 3 hours in the refrigerator.

- If using wooden skewers, soak for at least 30 minutes before grilling. This will help you avoid burning the wood.

- Rinse the tomatoes. Add the steak and tomatoes onto the skewers, alternating. Cook over a grill. Use the remaining marinating juices to baste. Use a meat thermometer if necessary to check the internal temperature of the beef (at least 165-170 degrees Fahrenheit).

- Serve immediately.

Chinese Orange Cabbage Wraps

This is a delicious and refreshing lunchtime option! The orange flavor pairs so well with the steak, adding a delightful touch of sweetness.

The following recipe counts as 1 serving of protein and 1 serving of vegetable.

Ingredients you will need for this recipe:

- Cabbage leaves (3-4, large)
- Lean steak, cut into strips (100 g)
- Vinegar (apple cider) (3 T.)
- Fresh minced garlic (2 cloves)
- Onion powder (0.25 t.)
- Ginger, grated (0.25 t.)
- Orange zest (1 orange)
- Orange juice (1 orange)
- Stevia, to taste
- Ground black peppercorns and sea salt, to taste

How to prepare this recipe:

- In a steamer or microwave, sprinkle the cabbage leaves with water and steam until tender. Remove and set aside.
- In a sauté pan or wok, add the steak, vinegar, garlic, onion powder, and ginger, and cook to a medium/high heat. Add the water in spoonfuls as necessary to prevent from sticking. Cook until steak is lightly browned.
- Add the rest of the ingredients. Cook the steak until browned and finished. Use a meat thermometer if necessary to check the internal temperature of the beef (at least 165-170 degrees Fahrenheit).
- To serve, wrap the steak in the cabbage leaves.

Quick Steak and Cauliflower Stir-Fry

This is a fantastic and quick stir-fry recipe to keep on hand for those weeknight dinners. The cauliflower in this recipe is phenomenal, and you can be glad that you're getting your serving of cruciferous vegetables for the day.

The following recipe counts as 1 serving of protein and 1 serving of vegetable.

Ingredients you will need for this recipe:

For the sauce:

- Liquid amino acids (0.5 T.)
- Lemon juice (0.25 T.)
- Water (0.5 T.)

For the steak:

- Lean steak, sliced into thin strips (100 g)
- Fresh minced garlic (0.5 t.)
- Ginger, grated (0.5 t.)
- Cauliflower, roughly chopped into small florets and stems (1 C.)
- Ground black peppercorns and sea salt, to taste

How to prepare this recipe:

- Combine the sauce ingredients in a small bowl. Set aside.
- Heat a large sauté pan or wok to a medium/high heat. Add the steak and salt and then add the water in spoonfuls as necessary to prevent from sticking. Stir occasionally until the steak is browned. Use a meat thermometer if necessary to check the

internal temperature of the beef (at least 165-170 degrees Fahrenheit).

- Remove the steak and set aside.

- Reduce the heat to medium and add the garlic and ginger. Add a spoonful of water. Stir for 30 seconds or when you start to smell the spices. Add the cauliflower and cook until tender (about 5 minutes). Add the water as necessary.

- Add the steak and liquid amino sauce mixture to the sauté pan. Stir until combined.

- Turn off the stovetop, transfer to a bowl, and serve.

Beef, Garlic, and Onion Kabobs

This grilled kabobs recipe highlights a number of delicious, classic flavors. Take note of the skewer's tip below if you're using wooden sticks. This will really help ensure that you don't end up with charred skewers.

The following recipe counts as 1 serving of protein and 1 serving of vegetable.

Ingredients you will need for this recipe:

- Lean steak, cubed (100 g)

- Onion, cut into 8 wedges (1 whole onion)

- Ground garlic (0.25 t.)

- Onion powder (0.25 t.)

- Ground black peppercorns and sea salt, to taste

How to prepare this recipe:

- In a bowl, combine the steak with the garlic powder and onion powder.

- If using wooden skewers, soak for at least 30 minutes before grilling. This will help you avoid burning the wood.

- Add the steak and onion onto the skewers, alternating. Top with sea salt and ground black peppercorns, if used.

- Cook over a grill. Use a meat thermometer if necessary to check the internal temperature of the beef (at least 165-170 degrees Fahrenheit).

- Serve immediately.

Spicy Kung Pao Shrimp

This shrimp recipe features that classic kung pao heat! Use dried Chinese red chili peppers if you can find them for true authenticity, but red pepper flakes make a great alternative. Adjust spice based on your tastes.

The following recipe counts as 1 serving of protein and 1 serving of vegetable.

Ingredients you will need for this recipe:

For the sauce:

- Liquid amino acids (1 T.)
- Water (2 T.)
- Ground white peppercorns (0.5 t.)
- Vinegar (apple cider) (0.25 t.)
- Stevia, to taste

For shrimp:

- Ginger, sliced (0.5 pieces)
- Water (2 T.)
- Onion, sliced (1 onion)
- Dried Chinese red chilies (5 whole) or red pepper flakes (0.5 T. or to taste)
- Shrimp (shelled, peeled, and deveined) (100 g)
- Sea salt to taste

How to prepare this recipe:

- Take a small bowl and mix the ingredients listed for the sauce. Set aside.

- Heat a large sauté pan or wok on medium heat. Add the ginger and stir a few times. Add spoonfuls of water as necessary to prevent sticking.

- Add the onion and red chilies (or red pepper flakes) and stir until fragrant.

- Add the shrimp and stir occasionally until cooked through. Lower the heat to medium and add the sauce. Mix until combined.

- Turn off the stovetop, transfer to a bowl, and serve immediately. Add the salt to taste.

Chinese Curried Shrimp

This is a simple and delicious recipe. Adjust curry powder levels based on your desired heat level!

The following recipe counts as 1 serving of protein and 1 serving of vegetable.

Ingredients you will need for this recipe:

- Onion, diced into 0.5-inch pieces (1 onion)
- Fresh minced garlic (3-4 cloves)
- Shrimp (100 g)
- Water (0.125 C.)
- Curry powder (0.5 t.)
- Ground cumin (0.5 t.)
- Red pepper flakes (0.25 t.)
- Ground black peppercorns and sea salt, to taste

How to prepare this recipe:

- Heat a sauté pan over medium heat.
- Add the onion and garlic. Add a spoonful of water if they begin to stick. Cook until they are fragrant and translucent.
- Add the shrimp, water, curry powder, cumin, red pepper flakes, salt, and pepper. Stir well to combine and stir-fry until the shrimps are opaque and fully cooked.

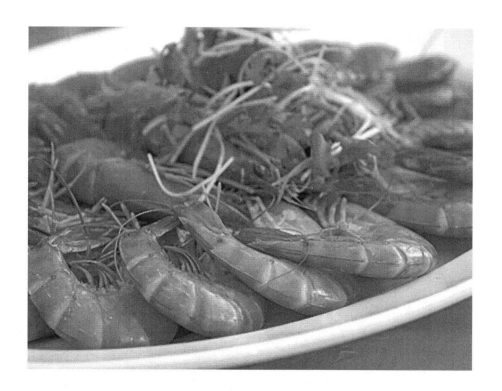

Cantonese Boiled Shrimp and Ginger Dipping Sauce

This is a classic Cantonese and Hong Kong dish heralded by many diners. It is simple, allowing the sweetness of the shrimp to stand out. Use fresh shrimp if you can; it makes all the difference.

The following recipe counts as 1 serving of protein and 1 serving of vegetable.

For the dipping sauce:

- Fresh finely grated ginger (0.5 T.)

- Liquid amino acids (0.5 T.)

- Water (0.25 T.)

- Green onions, minced (1 T.)

- Stevia, to taste

For shrimp:

- Water (approximately 2 C., just to cover shrimp)

- Ginger (1 slice)

- Green onion (1 whole)

- Sea salt (0.25 T.)

- Shrimp (shelled, peeled, and deveined) (100 g)

How to prepare this recipe:

- Prepare the sauce. Combine the ginger, liquid amino acids, water, and green onions in a small bowl. Add the stevia to taste.

- Add the 2 cups of water, ginger, green onion, and salt to a saucepan to a medium/high heat. Bring the water to a boil.

- Add all of the shrimps and stir slowly until they turn pink and begin floating. Turn off the stovetop, transfer to a bowl, and drain.

- Serve the shrimp immediately with the dipping sauce. Alternatively, chill in the refrigerator until ready to serve.

Cantonese-Style Steamed Sea Bass

This is another classic Cantonese dish, this time featuring a delicious ginger- and garlic-flavored sea bass fish. Traditionally, this dish was presented using a whole fish, plated and garnished to truly impress during important meals. Feel free to substitute other white fish for the sea bass specified.

The following recipe counts as 1 serving of protein and 1 serving of vegetable.

Ingredients you will need for this recipe:

For the fish:

- Water (2 C.)

- Sea bass fillets (can substitute other white fish) (100 g)

- Liquid amino acids (1 T.)

For the sauce:

- Vinegar (apple cider) (1 t.)

- Fresh minced garlic (2 cloves)

- Fresh finely grated ginger (1 T.)

- Green onions, thinly sliced (0.5 C.)

- Stevia, to taste

How to prepare this recipe:

- Place the fish in a steamer and cover and steam over boiling water for 10 to 15 minutes.

- Take a small bowl and combine the ingredients listed for the sauce.

- Look at the fish to see if it's fully cooked; the flesh should be white and mostly opaque.

- Remove the fish from the steamer and serve. First, pour the liquid amino acids over the fish and then the sauce.

Traditional Fish Casserole Stew

The casserole stew is a delicious, hearty, and warming dish found at many Chinese-American restaurants. This version uses fish, making it a slightly lighter take, but with all the requisite flavor.

The following recipe counts as 1 serving of protein and 1 serving of vegetable.

Ingredients you will need for this recipe:

- Whitefish fillets (100 g)

- Sea salt (0.25 t.)

- Vinegar (apple cider) (0.5 t.)

- Fresh finely grated ginger (0.5-inch piece)

- Dried Chinese red chilies (3 whole) or red pepper flakes (0.25 T. or to taste)

- Fresh minced garlic (2 cloves)

- Water (0.25 C., plus more as required)

- Liquid amino acids (0.5 T.)

- Stevia (1 packet)

- Ground white peppercorns (0.5 t.)

- Celery, cut into 1-inch lengths (1 C.)

How to prepare this recipe:

- In a bowl, marinate the fish fillets with the salt, vinegar, and half of the ginger for at least 30 minutes.

- Heat a wok or sauté pan over high heat until hot. Place the fish fillets into the pan with a few spoonfuls of water to prevent from sticking. Sauté with more water as required until lightly cooked. Take the fish out and set aside.

- To the pan, add the red chilies (or red pepper flakes), garlic, and the rest of the ginger. Cook until fragrant. Add spoonfuls of water as necessary to prevent from sticking and burning.

- Add the water, liquid amino acids, stevia, and ground white pepper to the pan, and bring to a boil. Return the fish to the pan as well and bring back to a boil.

- Put the celery in the pan and stir the mixture gently.

- Lower the heat to medium, cover the pan, and cook for a few more minutes just until the fish is well done and some of the water has cooked off.

- Turn off the stovetop, transfer to a bowl, and serve immediately. Add the salt and ground black peppercorns, to taste.

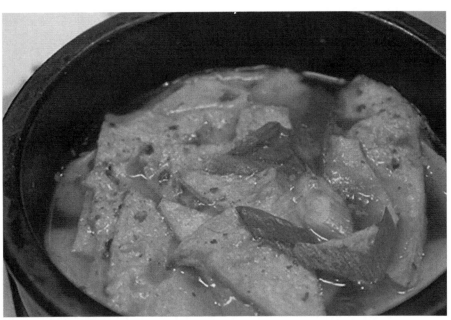

Chapter 6

Drinks and Desserts

Iced Herbal Chrysanthemum Tea

You can purchase chrysanthemum tea in tea bag form. The traditional Chinese way, however, is to use whole dried flowers. When placed in the water, they unfurl, blossoming and releasing a beautiful soft fragrance. This tea can also be taken hot if you prefer it that way.

Ingredients you will need for this recipe:

- Dried chrysanthemum flowers (1 T.)

- Water (1 C.)

- Stevia, to taste

How to prepare this recipe:

- Rinse the chrysanthemum flowers lightly.

- Allow the water to boil in a teapot.

- Add the flowers and keep at a simmer for 3-8 minutes, depending on preferred strength.

- Turn off the stovetop, transfer to a bowl, and strain. Traditionally, the chrysanthemum flowers are used repeatedly by adding more water to the pot. Each batch will get weaker, however.

- Add the, and stir to combine. Allow it to cool.

- Add the ice and serve chilled. Garnish with chrysanthemum flowers, if you desire.

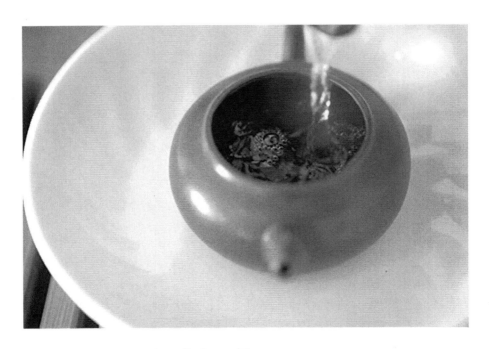

Metabolism-Boosting Oolong Tea

Oolong tea is well-known for boosting metabolism. You can purchase oolong tea in tea bag form. The traditional Chinese way, however, is to use whole oolong tea leaves directly in the teapot.

Ingredients you will need for this recipe:

- Dried oolong tea leaves (1 T.)

- Water (1 C.)

How to prepare this recipe:

- Rinse the oolong tea leaves lightly.

- Allow the water to boil in a teapot.

- Add the oolong tea and keep at a simmer for 3-5 minutes, depending on preferred strength.

- Turn off the stovetop, transfer to a bowl, and strain.

- Serve hot immediately.

Chinese Ginger Green Tea

Green tea is purported to have weight loss benefits. You can purchase green tea in tea bag form. The traditional Chinese way, however, is to use whole green tea leaves directly in the teapot.

Ingredients you will need for this recipe:

- Dried green tea leaves (1 T.)

- Water (1 C.)

- Ginger (1 slice)

- Stevia, optional, to taste

How to prepare this recipe:

- Rinse the green tea leaves lightly.

- Allow the water to boil in a teapot.

- Add the green tea and ginger and keep at a simmer for 1-3 minutes, depending on the preferred strength.

- Turn off the stovetop, transfer to a bowl, and strain.

- Add the stevia if used and mix to combine thoroughly.

- Serve hot immediately. You can also allow this to cool and drink chilled over ice.

Dim Sum Pu-er Tea

Pu-er is a classic tea that is often drank alongside dim sum. This is the perfect tea to serve with your Chinese-American meal. You can purchase pu-er tea in tea bag form. The traditional Chinese way, however, is to use whole pu-er tea leaves directly in the teapot.

Ingredients you will need for this recipe:

- Dried pu-er tea, either loose leaves or in a cake form (1 T.)

- Water (1 C.)

How to prepare this recipe:

- If using pu-er tea in a cake form, as it is commonly found, loosely tease the leaves apart from the cake. If the tea leaves are too compressed together, they will take longer to steep. Adjust steeping time if leaves are very tight together.

- Rinse the pu-er leaves lightly.

- Allow the water to boil in a teapot.

- Add the pu-er and keep at a simmer for 3-5 minutes, depending on preferred strength.

- Turn off the stovetop, transfer to a bowl, and strain. Traditionally, the pu-er tea leaves are used repeatedly by adding more water to the pot. Each batch will get weaker, however.

- Serve hot immediately.

Spiced Apple Cider

The Chinese 5-spices powder makes this a standout cider recipe! Enjoy on a cool night as an after dinner treat.

One cup of the following recipe counts as 1 serving of fruit.

Ingredients you will need for this recipe:

- Apples (4 whole)

- Water (5 C.)

- Stevia (4 packets)

- Cinnamon (1 t.)

- Chinese 5-spice powder (0.5 t.)

- Cinnamon stick (optional)

How to prepare this recipe:

- Peel and remove the core from the apple. Slice into large-sized slices.

- In a saucepan, place the sliced apples and cover with water. Add the stevia, cinnamon, and Chinese 5-spice powder.

- Simmer the mixture on medium heat for approximately 30 to 40 minutes. The apples should have softened and can be easily pierced and mushed with a fork.

- Remove the apples and save for separate use.

- Serve the cider immediately, with a cinnamon stick, if you desire.

- Store the remaining cider in the fridge for up to a week or freeze and thaw for an icy treat. Drink up to 1 cup a day.

Oranges With Ginger Simple Syrup

Fresh oranges get a sweet twist with spicy ginger simple syrup. Enjoy the ginger syrup over other fruits as well.

The following recipe counts as 1 serving of fruit.

Ingredients you will need for this recipe:

- Water (0.5 C.)

- Ginger (3 slices)

- Stevia (5 packets)

- Orange (1 whole)

- Chinese 5-spice powder (0.5 t.) (optional)

How to prepare this recipe:

- Allow the water to boil in a saucepan. Add the stevia and ginger slices. Simmer until the stevia has dissolved.

- Turn off the stovetop, transfer to a bowl, and allow to cool, preferably to room temperature.

- Peel the orange and slice or chop as desired.

- Drizzle the syrup to taste over the oranges. Reserve the remaining syrup for future use.

- Sprinkle with 5-spice powder, if you desire. Serve immediately.

Chinese Five-Spiced Applesauce

Applesauce is a healthy and hearty dessert. The Chinese 5-spices powder adds a slightly savory note, making this a great applesauce to pair alongside or after a heavy meat dish.

The following recipe counts as 1 serving of fruit.

Ingredients you will need for this recipe:

- Allspice berries (2)

- Cloves, whole (2)

- Fennel seed (0.125 T.)

- Whole black peppercorns (0.25 t.)

- Cinnamon stick (0.5 stick)

- Star anise (1)

- Apple, sweet variety (2 whole)

- Lemon juice (0.5 lemons)

- Stevia (1 packet)

- Sea salt (a pinch)

How to prepare this recipe:

- Preheat the oven to 350 degrees Fahrenheit.

- In a small piece of cheesecloth, bundle the allspice berries, cloves, fennel, whole peppercorns, cinnamon stick, and star anise. Use a piece of twine to tie off the cheesecloth into a small pouch.

- Peel and remove the core from the apple and slice into thin-sized slices.

- In a big Dutch oven, toss the apple slices with most of the lemon juice and the stevia. Reserve a tablespoon of the lemon juice for later.

- Heat the Dutch oven to medium/high heat, stirring once in a while, until the apples begin to lose moisture, approximately 5 minutes.

- Add the spice bundle to the pot. Put a lid on it and then move it to the preheated oven. Bake for approximately 1 hour and 30 minutes. Check occasionally and remove when the apples have softened enough to be fully mashed.

- Remove and discard the bundle of spices. Add the last tablespoon of lemon juice to the apple mixture and season with salt to taste. Stir with a large wooden spoon until the chunky sauce forms.

- Serve warm immediately. Alternatively, allow to cool, preferably to room temperature, and refrigerate in an airtight container for up to a week.

Traditional Restaurant Orange Slices

Traditional Chinese-American restaurants serve orange slices at the end of the meal. It's a healthy and sweet way to finish the night, symbolizing luck and prosperity.

The following recipe counts as 1 serving of fruit.

Ingredients you will need for this recipe:

- Orange (1 whole)

- Lemon juice, to taste

- Stevia, to taste

How to prepare this recipe:

- Wash the orange. Keep the peel on.

- Slice perpendicular to the blossom/navel.

- Arrange in a circle on a plate and sprinkle the lemon juice and stevia on top.

- Serve immediately.

Boiled Chinese Ginger Apples

Enjoy this simple but sweet recipe and satisfy your sweet tooth! Apples provide a great source of fiber, and ginger and cinnamon provide a delightful touch of spice.

The following recipe counts as 1 serving of fruit.

Ingredients you will need for this recipe:

- Apple (1 whole)
- Ginger (1 t.)
- Cinnamon (1 t.)
- Stevia (1 package)
- Water (1 C.)

How to prepare this recipe:

- Remove the core from the apple and slice into medium-sized slices.
- Place the apple slices and all other ingredients into a saucepan. Cook on high heat until boiling.

Index

Recipes by the Main Ingredient

List of Vegetable Recipes

List of Rice Recipes

Simple Egg Fried Rice

List of Egg Recipes

Classic Egg Drop Soup

Simple Egg Fried Rice

List of Beef Recipes

Ginger Beef Stew

Cabbage and Beef Soup

Beef Egg Roll Bowl

Beef Konjac Chow Fun Noodles

Ginger Beef and Onions

Healthy Beef and Broccoli

Ginger Steak and Tomato Skewers

Orange Cabbage Wraps

Quick Steak and Cauliflower Stir-Fry

Beef, Garlic, and Onion Kabobs

List of Chicken Recipes

Chinese Chicken and Broccoli Soup

Simple Curry Chicken Soup

Asparagus and Chicken Salad With Ginger Dressing

Easy Chicken Broth

Easy Orange Chicken

General Tso's Chicken

Orange Chicken Wraps

Dim Sum Chicken Meatballs

Classic Chicken Stir-Fry

Simple Garlic Chicken

Low-Fat Sweet and Sour Chicken

List of Shrimp Recipes

Spicy Kung Pao Shrimp

Chinese Curried Shrimp

Cantonese Boiled Shrimp and Ginger Dipping Sauce

List of Fish Recipes

Banquet Imitation Shark Fin Soup

Cantonese-Style Steamed Sea Bass

Traditional Fish Casserole Stew

List of Tea Recipes

Iced Herbal Chrysanthemum Tea

Metabolism-Boosting Oolong Tea

Ginger Green Tea

Dim Sum Pu-er Tea

List of Fruit Recipes

Spiced Apple Cider

Oranges With Ginger Simple Syrup

Chinese Five-Spiced Applesauce

Traditional Restaurant Orange Slices

Boiled Chinese Ginger Apples

Conclusion

I hope this book was able to help you discover the joy in cooking delicious, HCG-friendly, Chinese-American dishes.

The next step in losing weight is to keep making these delicious, simple recipes. Consider these as the basis for your own creativity; tweak the recipe's ingredients based on the seasons or what's on sale while adhering to the restrictions of the HCG protocol. The beauty of cooking lies in the creative potential, and if you can enjoy the process of cooking, it will be all the easier to make meals for yourself rather than buying unhealthy prepackaged, processed foods. Now that you know how easy it is to make your own food, you won't need to order Chinese takeout next week!

Most importantly, believe in your ability to stick with the HCG diet plan. Commit yourself to following the guidelines, as difficult as it may seem, and you will see results. As your body realizes that it does not need as many calories, sugar, or salt as it was consuming before, it will grow to love nutritious food and the amazing way that it can make you feel. It's important to remember that eating well is a lifelong strategy. Any dieting strategy should be thoroughly reviewed with your physician, but hopefully, these recipes have helped you understand how simple it can be to eat well and lose weight.

If you enjoyed this book, it would be much appreciated if you could leave a good review for it on Amazon.

Thanks, and I wish you luck!

Made in the USA
Columbia, SC
23 January 2021

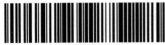